SUPER EASY TYPE 2 DIABETES COOKBOOK FOR BEGINNERS 2024

1500 Days of Super Easy, Tasty and Delicious Low Sugar & Low-Carb Recipes to Manage Type 2 Diabetes with 28-Days Meal Plan

TERESA R. THOMAS

Table of Contents

INTRODUCTION

My doctor suggested a simple blood test when I was 35 years old, which indicated that I had Type 2 diabetes. My parents both had type 2 diabetes; my mother was diagnosed when she was 30 and my father in his mid-40s.

Having said that, almost everyone on the earth has met or heard of someone with diabetes, whether it's a friend or family. When you are diagnosed with type 2 diabetes, you must adopt lifestyle modifications to be healthy.

I can confirm that it hasn't always been easy; there have been several obstacles to overcome. I can honestly say that eating healthily has improved my life.

Going on this life-changing path may be intimidating since you are expected to drastically modify your eating habits, which may be difficult for those who have just been diagnosed with type 2 diabetes.

You quickly understand that if you don't manage your type 2 diabetes properly, you risk developing heart disease, chronic kidney disease, nerve damage, and other foot, dental, vision, hearing, and mental health issues.

Throughout this book, I'll provide specific diabetic-friendly recipes that have worked for me over the years, as well as which foods are best and worst for diabetes. I've included a meal plan to help you plan all of your diabetic meals. I've also included a list of dietary foods that may help you manage Type 2 diabetes, as well as suggestions for managing and treating the condition.

We'll go over the types of diabetes, what they are, and what you should do if you believe you have diabetic symptoms.

If you unexpectedly develop diabetes symptoms or come into touch with someone who does, this book is all you'll need.

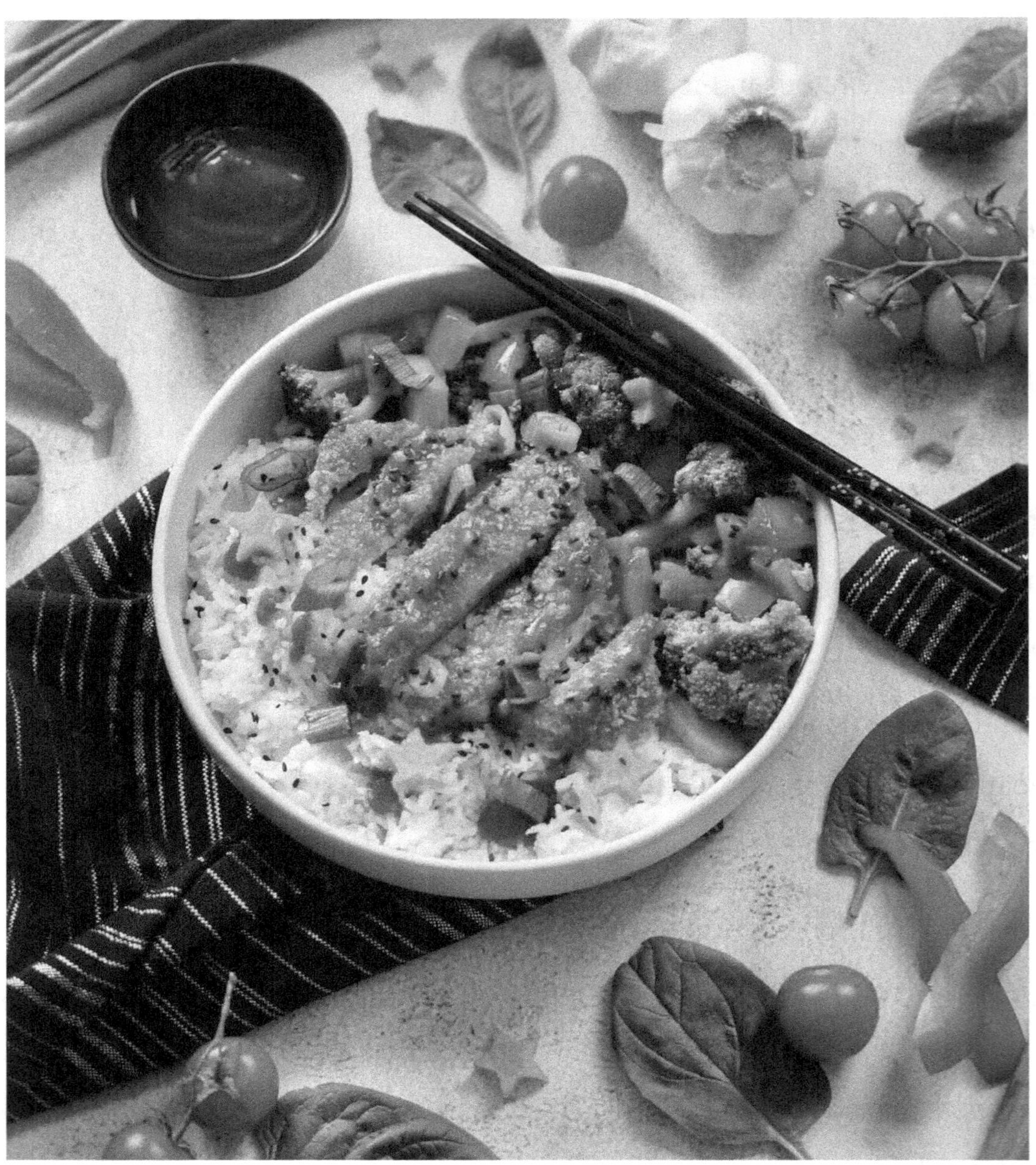

CHAPTER 1

What is Type 2 Diabetes?

Type 2 diabetes is a chronic medical disorder in which sugar, or glucose, accumulates in the circulation. This occurs when your body is unable to efficiently respond to insulin or produces insufficient amounts of it.

Typically, insulin helps transfer glucose from your blood to your cells, where it is utilized for energy. However, with type 2 diabetes, your body's cells are unable to react to insulin as well as they should. In the latter stages of the illness, your body may not create enough insulin.

Uncontrolled type 2 diabetes may result in persistently high blood glucose levels, causing a variety of symptoms and possibly dangerous consequences.

Symptoms of Type 2 Diabetes

In type 2 diabetes, your body is unable to efficiently utilize insulin to transport glucose into your cells. This forces your body to depend on other energy sources in your tissues, muscles, and organs. This is a chain reaction that may induce a wide range of symptoms.

Type 2 diabetes may progress slowly. The symptoms may be modest and easily dismissed at first. Early signs may include:

Symptoms may include:

- Constant hunger

- Low Energy and Weariness.

- Extreme thirst and frequent urination.

- Blurred vision.

- Numbness, tingling, or discomfort in the hands or feet.

As the condition advances, the symptoms worsen and may lead to serious problems.

Complications of having high blood glucose levels over an extended period may include:

- Eye issues (including diabetic retinopathy).

- Numbness in the extremities, also known as neuropathy.

- Nephropathy (kidney disease).

- Gum disease.

- Heart attack or stroke.

Causes of Type 2 Diabetes

Insulin is a naturally occurring hormone. Your pancreas makes and secretes it when you eat. Insulin transports glucose from the circulation to cells throughout your body, where it is converted into energy.

If you have type 2 diabetes, your body becomes insulin-resistant. Your body is no longer able to adequately use the hormone. This makes your pancreas work harder to produce more insulin.

This may eventually cause pancreatic cell destruction. Eventually, your pancreas may be unable to make insulin.

If you don't create enough insulin or your body doesn't utilize it properly, glucose accumulates in your bloodstream. This depletes your body's energy reserves. Doctors aren't sure what causes this string of occurrences. It might be due to pancreatic cell malfunction or cell signaling and regulation.

While type 2 diabetes is mostly caused by lifestyle decisions, you may be more likely to be diagnosed if:

- Your family history suggests a genetic propensity to type 2 diabetes.

- Your family has a hereditary propensity to fat, which raises the risk of insulin resistance and diabetes.

- You're at least 45 years old.

- You are Black, Hispanic/Latino, Native American, or of Alaska Native origin.

While your body's resistance to insulin is the definitive cause of type 2 diabetes, a combination of variables often increases your likelihood of developing that resistance.

Treatment for Type 2 Diabetes

Type 2 diabetes is manageable and, in some situations, reversible. Most treatment programs will entail measuring your blood glucose levels, and your doctor will advise you on how often you should do it. The objective is to remain inside a certain range.

Your doctor will most likely recommend the following lifestyle adjustments to help manage your type 2 diabetes:

- Eating fiber-rich foods and healthy carbs, such as fruits, vegetables, and whole grains, may help maintain stable blood glucose levels.

- Eat at regular intervals.

- Learning to listen to your body and quit eating when you're satisfied.

- Maintain a healthy weight and heart by limiting your intake of processed carbs, sweets, and animal fats.

- Get around 30 minutes of physical activity every day to help keep your heart healthy; exercise may also help lower blood glucose levels.

Your doctor will explain how to spot early signs of high or low blood sugar and what to do in each case.

Working with a dietitian may also help you understand which meals can help you regulate your blood sugar and which might cause it to become imbalanced.

Not everyone with type 2 diabetes has to take insulin. If you do, it's because your pancreas isn't producing enough insulin on its own, and you should take insulin as prescribed. Other prescription drugs may also help.

Medications for Type 2 Diabetes

In some situations, lifestyle adjustments are sufficient to keep type 2 diabetes under control. If not, there are a few drugs that might assist. Some of these drugs are:

- **Metformin:** This medication may reduce blood glucose levels and enhance your body's response to insulin. It is the first-line therapy for the majority of persons with type 2 diabetes.

- **Sulfonylureas** are oral drugs that assist your body produce more insulin.

- **Meglitinides:** These are short-acting drugs that cause your pancreas to produce more insulin.

- **Thiazolidinediones:** These help your body respond to insulin.

- **DPP-4 inhibitors:** These are gentler drugs that lower blood glucose levels.

- **Glucagon-like peptide-1 agonists**: These reduce digestion and raise blood sugar levels.

- **Sodium-glucose Cotransporter-2 (SGLT2) Inhibitors:** These assist your kidneys to eliminate sugar from your body via urine.

Each of the medications mentioned above may induce negative effects. It may take some time for you and your doctor to determine the most effective drug or combination of medicines to manage diabetes.

If your blood pressure or cholesterol levels are not optimal, you may need drugs to treat those issues as well.

If your body is unable to produce enough insulin, you may need insulin treatment. You may simply need a long-acting injection to take at night, or you may need to take insulin numerous times each day.

Diet for Type 2 Diabetes

Diet is a key strategy for maintaining good heart health and blood glucose levels that are within acceptable limits.

The diet suggested for persons with type 2 diabetes is the same one that most people should follow. It comes down to a few main actions:

- Select a range of meals that are rich in nutrients yet low in empty calories.

- Practice being conscious of portion sizes and quitting eating when you are full.

- Read food labels carefully to see how much sugar or carbohydrates you may be consuming in a single serving.

Foods and Drinks to be Limited

If you have type 2 diabetes, or if you want to prevent diabetes and maintain your weight, you should restrict certain meals and drinks. This includes:

- Foods rich in saturated and Trans fats (such as red meat and full-fat dairy products).

- Processed meats like hot dogs and salami.

- Refined baked foods, such as white bread and cake, may include margarine and shortening

- High-sugar, highly processed foods (packaged cookies and some cereals)

- Sugary beverages (such as ordinary soda and some fruit juices)

While no one meal should derail you from your healthy lifestyle, you should see your doctor about dietary limits depending on your blood sugar levels. Some individuals may need to check their glucose levels more closely than others after consuming these items.

Food to Choose

Being diagnosed with type 2 diabetes does not imply you can't eat carbohydrates. Healthy carbs may give you both energy and fiber. Some choices are:

- Whole fruits.

- Non-starchy veggies, such as broccoli, carrots, and cauliflower.

- Legumes, such as beans, and whole grains, such as oats or quinoa.

- Sweet potatoes

Fat is not off the menu either. Instead, it's about selecting the correct kinds of fat. The following foods contain heart-healthy omega-3 fatty acids:

- Tuna, sardines, salmon, mackerel, halibut, cod, and flax seeds.

- Many foods contain healthful monounsaturated and polyunsaturated fats, such as:

- Oils, including olive oil

- Nuts, including almonds, pecans, and walnuts

- Avocados

Talk to your doctor about your particular dietary objectives. They may propose that you consult with a dietitian who specializes in diabetes-friendly foods. Together, you can create a diet plan that tastes wonderful and meets your lifestyle requirements.

Risk Factors for Type 2 Diabetes

While certain risk factors for Type 2 diabetes are beyond your control (such as your age and background, as previously stated), some lifestyle decisions may also increase your chance of getting type 2 diabetes. Some of them include:

- Being overweight: Being overweight increases the amount of fatty tissue in your body, making your cells more resistant to insulin.

- Living a more sedentary lifestyle: Regular physical exercise improves insulin sensitivity.

- Consuming a lot of highly processed food. Highly processed meals may include a lot of hidden sugar and refined carbohydrates. If your lifestyle necessitates a more "grab-and-go" eating habit, see your doctor or a nutritionist about healthful alternatives.

You may also be at a higher risk if you have gestational diabetes or prediabetes, both of which are characterized by high blood glucose levels.

Tips for Preventing Type 2 Diabetes

While type 2 diabetes cannot always be prevented, there are a few lifestyle changes that may help postpone or even prevent its development. This is true even if you have higher risk factors, such as pre-diabetes.

- **Diet:** The optimal diet for preventing type 2 diabetes is one high in fruits and vegetables, healthy carbohydrates and fats, and low in processed sugars.

- **Exercise:** According to the 2018 Physical Activity Guidelines for Americans, the recommended amount of exercise per week for adults is 150 minutes, which translates to 30 minutes per day, 5 days per week. The Physical Activities Guidelines also advocate a mix of muscular strength and aerobic activities.

- **Weight management:** Maintaining a reasonable weight might help you prevent chronic issues like type 2 diabetes.

Complications Associated With Type 2 Diabetes

Many individuals may properly control their type 2 diabetes. If not adequately controlled, it may damage almost all of your organs and cause major consequences, including:

- Skin issues, such as bacterial or fungal infections.

- Nerve damage, also known as neuropathy, may cause loss of feeling, numbness, and tingling in your extremities, as well as digestive problems such as vomiting, diarrhea, and constipation.

- Poor circulation to the feet, making it difficult for your feet to recover when you have a cut or an infection, and may potentially lead to gangrene and loss of the foot or limb.

- Hearing impairment.

- Retinal damage, or retinopathy, and eye damage, which may result in poor eyesight, glaucoma, and cataracts.

- Cardiovascular illnesses such as excessive blood pressure, arterial narrowing, angina, heart attack, and stroke.

- Those with diabetes are more likely to have a heart attack at a younger age than those without diabetes.

- Men with diabetes are 3.5 times more likely to have Erectile Dysfunction (ED).

Managing Type 2 Diabetes

Managing type 2 diabetes involves collaboration. You'll need to work closely with your doctor, but your decisions will have a significant impact on the outcome.

Your doctor may recommend frequent blood tests to determine your blood glucose levels. This will assist assess how effectively you're handling the situation. If you take medicine, these tests can help you determine how effectively it works.

Your doctor may also offer home monitoring equipment that allows you to test your blood glucose levels in between appointments. They will tell you how frequently you should use it and what your goal range should be.

Diabetes may raise your risk of cardiovascular disease, so your doctor may want to check your blood pressure and cholesterol levels. If you experience signs of heart disease, you may need more testing. These tests may involve an electrocardiogram (ECG or EKG) or a heart stress test.

It may also be beneficial to include your family in the process. Educating children about the warning symptoms of abnormally high or low blood glucose levels can enable them to assist in an emergency.

CHAPTER 2

1. Zucchini Fritters

Ingredients:

- 2 medium zucchinis, grated

- 1/4 cup grated Parmesan cheese

- 1/4 cup all-purpose flour

- 1 egg, beaten

- 2 cloves garlic, minced

- Salt and pepper to taste

- Olive oil for frying

Preparation:

1. Grate the zucchini and squeeze out excess moisture using a clean kitchen towel.

2. In a bowl, combine the grated zucchini, Parmesan cheese, flour, beaten egg, minced garlic, salt, and pepper.

3. Heat olive oil in a skillet over medium heat.

4. Scoop spoonful of the zucchini mixture onto the skillet, flattening them into patties.

5. Cook until golden brown on both sides, about 3-4 minutes per side.

6. Serve hot with your favorite dipping sauce or yogurt.

Nutritional Value: Each serving contains approximately 120 calories, 6g fat, 10g carbohydrates, and 6g protein.

Cooking Time: About 20 minutes
Number of Servings: Makes 4 servings.

2. Tofu Scramble

Ingredients:

- Crumble one block of super firm tofu.

- 1 tablespoon olive oil

- 1/2 onion, diced

- 1 bell pepper, diced

- 2 cups spinach

- 2 cloves garlic, minced

- 1/2 teaspoon turmeric

- Salt and pepper to taste

Preparation:

1. In a pan, heat the olive oil over a medium-high heat. Sauté the chopped onion and bell pepper until they soften.

2. Add minced garlic and crumbled tofu to the skillet. Cook for 5-7 minutes, stirring occasionally.

3. Sprinkle turmeric over the tofu mixture, and stir to combine. Season with salt and pepper.

4. Add spinach to the skillet and cook until wilted.

5. Serve hot with whole-grain toast or tortillas.

Nutritional Value: Each serving contains approximately 150 calories, 10g fat, 7g carbohydrates, 12g protein.

Cooking Time: About 15 minutes
Servings: Makes two.

3. Sweet Potato Hash

Ingredients:

- Peel and dice two medium sweet potatoes.

- 1 onion, diced

- 1 red bell pepper, diced

- 2 tablespoons olive oil

- 1 teaspoon smoked paprika

- 1/2 teaspoon garlic powder

- Salt and pepper to taste

Preparation:

1. In a pan, heat the olive oil over a medium-high heat. Add diced sweet potatoes and cook until slightly tender, about 8-10 minutes.

2. Add diced onion and red bell pepper to the skillet. Cook until vegetables are softened.

3. Sprinkle smoked paprika, garlic powder, salt, and pepper over the sweet potato mixture. Stir to combine.

4. Continue cooking until sweet potatoes are fully cooked and slightly caramelized.

5. Serve hot as a side dish or topped with a fried egg.

Nutritional Value: Each serving contains approximately 180 calories, 7g fat, 28g carbohydrates, 3g protein.

Cooking Time: About 20 minutes

Number of Servings: Makes 4 servings.

4. Egg and Veggie Skewers

Ingredients:

- 4 eggs

- 1 bell pepper, diced

- 1 zucchini, diced

- 1 cup cherry tomatoes

- Salt and pepper to taste

- Wooden skewers, soaked in water

Preparation:

1. Hard-boil the eggs, peel, and set aside to cool.

2. Thread diced bell pepper, zucchini, cherry tomatoes, and peeled hard-boiled eggs onto the skewers.

3. Sprinkle the skewers with salt and pepper.

4. Grill or broil the skewers until vegetables are tender and slightly charred.

5. Serve hot with your favorite dipping sauce or salsa.

Nutritional Value: Each serving contains approximately 130 calories, 6g fat, 10g carbohydrates, and 10g protein.

Cooking Time: About 15 minutes

Number of Servings: Makes 4 skewers.

5. Cauliflower Hash Browns

Ingredients:

- 1 small head cauliflower, grated or finely chopped

- 1/4 cup grated Parmesan cheese

- 1/4 cup almond flour

- 1 egg, beaten

- 1/2 teaspoon garlic powder

- Salt and pepper to taste

- Olive oil for frying

Preparation:

1. Place the grated cauliflower in a clean kitchen towel and squeeze out excess moisture.

2. In a bowl, combine the squeezed cauliflower, grated Parmesan cheese, almond flour, beaten egg, garlic powder, salt, and pepper.

3. Heat olive oil in a skillet over medium heat.

4. Scoop spoonful of the cauliflower mixture onto the skillet, flattening them into patties.

5. Cook until golden brown on both sides, about 3-4 minutes per side.

6. Serve hot with a dollop of Greek yogurt or salsa.

Nutritional Value: Each serving contains approximately 90 calories, 6g fat, 6g carbohydrates, and 4g protein.

Cooking Time: About 15 minutes

Number of Servings: Makes 4 servings.

6. Smoked Salmon Wrap

Ingredients:

- 4 whole wheat tortillas

- 4 oz smoked salmon

- 1/2 cup cream cheese

- 1 cucumber, thinly sliced

- 1 avocado, sliced

- Handful of arugula

- Salt and pepper to taste

Preparation:

1. Spread cream cheese equally on each tortilla.

2. Layer smoked salmon, cucumber slices, avocado slices, and arugula on each tortilla.

3. Add salt and pepper to taste.

4. Roll up the tortillas tightly, slice in half, and serve immediately.

Nutritional Value: Each serving contains approximately 300 calories, 15g fat, 30g carbohydrates, 15g protein.

Preparation Time: About 10 minutes

Number of Servings: Makes 4 wraps.

7. Chia Seed Pudding

Ingredients:

- 1/4 cup chia seeds

- 1 cup almond milk (or any milk of your choice)

- One tablespoon of maple sugar or honey.

- 1/2 teaspoon vanilla extract

- Fresh fruits or nuts for topping (optional)

Preparation:

1. In a bowl or jar, mix chia seeds, almond milk, maple syrup, and vanilla extract.

2. Stir well to combine and break up any clumps of chia seeds.

3. Cover and refrigerate for at least 2 hours, or overnight, until the mixture thickens and becomes pudding-like.

4. Stir the pudding before serving and add your favorite toppings such as fresh fruits or nuts.

Nutritional Value: Each serving contains approximately 150 calories, 8g fat, 15g carbohydrates, 6g protein.

Preparation time: around 5 minutes (plus chilling time).

Servings: 2

8. Quinoa Breakfast Bowl

Ingredients:

- 1 cup cooked quinoa

- 1/2 cup Greek yogurt

- 1 tablespoon of honey or maple syrup.

- 1/4 cup mixed berries (strawberries, blueberries, and raspberries)

- 1 tablespoon chopped nuts (such as almonds, and walnuts)

- 1 tablespoon unsweetened shredded coconut

- Cinnamon for sprinkling (optional)

Preparation:

1. In a bowl, layer cooked quinoa, Greek yogurt, mixed berries, chopped nuts, and shredded coconut.

2. Splash honey or maple syrup over top.

3. Sprinkle with cinnamon if desired.

4. Serve immediately and enjoy!

Nutritional Value: Each serving contains approximately 350 calories, 12g fat, 45g carbohydrates, 15g protein.

Preparation Time: About 10 minutes

Number of Servings: Makes 1 serving.

CHAPTER 3

1. Cauliflower Potato Salad

Ingredients:

- Cut a single medium-sized head of cauliflower into florets.

- 3 medium potatoes, boiled and diced

- 1/2 cup mayonnaise

- 2 tablespoons Dijon mustard

- 2 tablespoons apple cider vinegar

- 1/2 cup diced celery

- 1/4 cup diced red onion

- Salt and pepper to taste

Preparation:

1. Steam the cauliflower florets until tender, about 5-7 minutes. Let them cool.

2. In a large bowl, mix mayonnaise, Dijon mustard, and apple cider vinegar.

3. Add cauliflower, potatoes, celery, and red onion to the bowl. Mix until well combined.

4. Add salt and pepper to taste.

5. Chill for at least an hour before serving to enable the flavors to combine.

Nutritional Value: This recipe serves 4 and provides approximately 250 calories per serving.

2. Chicken Caesar Salad

Ingredients:

- 2 boneless, skinless chicken breasts

- Salt and pepper to taste

- 1 tablespoon olive oil

- 1 head romaine lettuce, chopped

- 1/2 cup Caesar dressing

- 1/4 cup grated Parmesan cheese

- 1 cup croutons

Preparation:

1. Season the chicken breasts with salt and pepper.

2. In a pan, heat the olive oil over medium heat. Cook the chicken breasts for 6-7 minutes on each side, or until well done.

3. Allow the chicken to rest for a few minutes before slicing it into strips.

4. In a large bowl, toss together romaine lettuce, Caesar dressing, Parmesan cheese, and croutons.

5. Top with sliced chicken and serve immediately.

Nutritional Value: This recipe serves 2 and provides approximately 400 calories per serving.

3. Spinach Strawberry Salad

Ingredients:

- 6 cups fresh spinach leaves

- 1 1/2 cups sliced strawberries

- 1/4 cup crumbled feta cheese

- 1/4 cup sliced almonds

- 2 tablespoons balsamic vinegar

- 1 tablespoon honey

- 2 tablespoons olive oil

- Salt and pepper to taste

Preparation:

1. In a large mixing bowl, add spinach, cut strawberries, feta cheese, and almonds.

2. In a small bowl, whisk together balsamic vinegar, honey, olive oil, salt, and pepper to make the dressing.

3. Pour the dressing over the salad and toss to coat evenly.

4. Serve immediately.

Nutritional Value: This recipe serves 4 and provides approximately 150 calories per serving.

4. Quinoa Chickpea Salad

Ingredients:

- 1 cup quinoa, rinsed

- 1 can (15 oz) chickpeas, drained and rinsed

- 1 red bell pepper, diced

- 1 cucumber, diced

- 1/4 cup chopped fresh parsley

- 1/4 cup chopped fresh mint

- 1/4 cup olive oil

- 2 tablespoons lemon juice

- Salt and pepper to taste

Preparation:

1. Cook quinoa according to package instructions. Let it cool.

2. In a large bowl, combine cooked quinoa, chickpeas, diced red bell pepper, diced cucumber, chopped parsley, and chopped mint.

3. In a small bowl, whisk together olive oil, lemon juice, salt, and pepper to make the dressing.

4. Pour the dressing over the salad and toss to coat evenly.

5. Serve chilled or at room temperature.

Nutritional Value: This recipe serves 4 and provides approximately 300 calories per serving.

5. Greek Cucumber Salad

Ingredients:

- 2 large cucumbers, diced
- 1 cup cherry tomatoes, halved
- 1/2 cup diced red onion
- 1/2 cup crumbled feta cheese
- 1/4 cup chopped fresh parsley
- 2 tablespoons olive oil
- 1 tablespoon red wine vinegar
- 1 teaspoon dried oregano
- Salt and pepper to taste

Preparation:

1. In a large bowl, combine diced cucumbers, cherry tomatoes, diced red onion, crumbled feta cheese, and chopped parsley.

2. In a small mixing bowl, combine the olive oil, red wine vinegar, dried oregano, salt, and pepper to prepare the dressing.

3. Pour the dressing over the salad and toss to coat evenly.

4. Serve chilled.

Nutritional Value: This recipe serves 4 and provides approximately 150 calories per serving.

6. Citrus Shrimp Salad

Ingredients:

- 1 lb peeled and deveined big shrimp

- 2 oranges zest and juice

- Zest and juice from 1 lemon.

- 2 tablespoons olive oil

- 2 cloves garlic, minced

- Salt and pepper to taste

- 6 cups mixed salad greens

- 1 avocado, diced

- 1/4 cup chopped fresh cilantro

Preparation:

1. In a large bowl, whisk together orange zest, orange juice, lemon zest, lemon juice, olive oil, minced garlic, salt, and pepper to make the marinade.

2. Add shrimp to the marinade and toss to coat. Let it marinate for 15-30 minutes.

3. Heat a skillet over medium-high heat. Cook shrimp for 2-3 minutes per side or until pink and cooked through.

4. In a large serving bowl, arrange mixed salad greens. Top with cooked shrimp, diced avocado, and chopped cilantro.

5. Serve immediately.

- Nutritional Value: This recipe serves 4 and provides approximately 250 calories per serving.

7. Watermelon Mint Salad

Ingredients:

- 4 cups diced seedless watermelon

- 1/4 cup crumbled feta cheese.

- 1/4 cup freshly cut mint leaves.

- 2 tablespoons balsamic glaze

Preparation:

1. In a large bowl, combine diced watermelon and chopped mint leaves.

2. Sprinkle crumbled feta cheese over the watermelon and mint.

3. Drizzle balsamic glaze over the salad.

4. Gently toss to combine.

5. Serve chilled.

Nutritional Value: This recipe serves 4 and provides approximately 100 calories per serving.

8. Tuna Avocado Salad

Ingredients:

- 2 cans (5 oz each) of tuna, drained

- 2 ripe avocados, diced

- 1/4 cup diced red onion

- 1/4 cup chopped fresh cilantro

- Juice of 1 lime

- Salt and pepper to taste

Preparation:

1. In a large bowl, combine drained tuna, diced avocado, diced red onion, chopped cilantro, and lime juice.

2. Season with salt and pepper to taste.

3. Gently toss to combine.

4. Serve immediately or chill until ready to serve.

Nutritional Value: This recipe serves 2 and provides approximately 300 calories per serving.

CHAPTER 4

1. Two Cheese Cauliflower

Ingredients:

- 1 head cauliflower, cut into florets

- 1 cup shredded cheddar cheese

- 1/2 cup grated Parmesan cheese

- 1/4 cup heavy cream

- Salt and pepper to taste

Preparation:

1. Preheat your oven to 375°F (190°C).

2. Steam the cauliflower florets until tender, about 5-7 minutes. Drain well.

3. In a mixing bowl, combine the steamed cauliflower, cheddar cheese, Parmesan cheese, heavy cream, salt, and pepper. Mix until well combined.

4. Transfer the mixture to a baking dish and distribute evenly.

5. Bake in the preheated oven for 20-25 minutes, or until the cheese melts and bubbles.

6. Serve hot and enjoy!

Nutritional Value (per serving):

- Calories: 250

- Total Fat: 18g

- Saturated Fat: 11g

- Cholesterol: 55mg

- Sodium: 400mg

- Total Carbohydrates: 10g

- Dietary Fiber: 3g

- Sugars: 3g

- Protein: 15g

Cooking Time: 30-35 minutes

Number of Servings: 4

2. Lemon-Herb Zucchini

Ingredients:

- Slice 4 medium zucchinis into rounds.

- 2 tablespoons olive oil

- 2 cloves garlic, minced

- Zest of 1 lemon

- Juice of 1 lemon

- 1 tablespoon chopped fresh parsley

- Salt and pepper to taste

Preparation:

1. Warm the olive oil in a large pan over medium heat.

2. Add the minced garlic and simmer for 1-2 minutes, until aromatic.

3. Add the zucchini slices to the skillet and cook for 5-7 minutes, stirring occasionally, until they are tender.

4. Add the lemon zest, lemon juice, chopped parsley, salt, and pepper to the skillet. Stir to mix, then simmer for another 1-2 minutes.

5. Remove from the fire and serve hot.

Nutritional Value (per serving):

- Calories: 80

- Total Fat: 6g

- Saturated Fat: 1g

- Sodium: 10mg

- Total Carbohydrates: 6g

- Dietary Fiber: 2g

- Sugars: 3g

- Protein: 2g

Cooking Time: 10-15 minutes

Number of Servings: 4

3. Cumin Mushrooms

Ingredients:

- 1 pound mushrooms, sliced

- 2 tablespoons olive oil

- 2 teaspoons ground cumin

- 2 cloves garlic, minced

- Salt and pepper to taste

- Fresh cilantro for garnish (optional)

Preparation:

1. Warm the olive oil in a pan over medium heat.

2. Add the minced garlic and cook for 1 minute until fragrant.

3. Add the sliced mushrooms to the skillet and cook for 5-7 minutes, stirring occasionally, until they are tender and browned.

4. Sprinkle the ground cumin over the mushrooms and stir to combine. Cook for an additional 1-2 minutes.

5. Add salt and pepper to taste.

6. Garnish with fresh cilantro if desired and serve hot.

Nutritional Value (per serving):

- Calories: 70

- Total Fat: 5g

- Saturated Fat: 1g

- Sodium: 5mg

- Total Carbohydrates: 5g

- Dietary Fiber: 2g

- Sugars: 2g

- Protein: 3g

Cooking Time: 10-15 minutes

Number of Servings: 4

4. Asparagus with Curried Walnut Butter

Ingredients:

- 1 pound asparagus, trimmed

- 1/4 cup walnuts, chopped

- 2 tablespoons unsalted butter

- 1 teaspoon curry powder

- Salt and pepper to taste

Preparation:

1. Steam or blanch the asparagus until tender, about 3-5 minutes. Drain and set aside.

2. In a small skillet, toast the chopped walnuts over medium heat for 2-3 minutes until fragrant. Remove from heat and set aside.

3. In the same skillet, heat the butter over low heat. Stir in the curry powder for approximately 1 minute, or until it is aromatic.

4. Add the toasted walnuts to the skillet with the butter and curry mixture. Stir to combine.

5. Arrange the steamed asparagus on a serving plate and drizzle the curried walnut butter over the top.

6. Add salt and pepper to taste.

7. Serve immediately.

Nutritional Value (per serving):

- Calories: 150

- Total Fat: 13g

- Saturated Fat: 4g

- Sodium: 60mg

- Total Carbohydrates: 6g

- Dietary Fiber: 3g

- Sugars: 2g

- Protein: 4g

Cooking Time: 10-15 minutes

Number of Servings: 4

5. Mushroom Risotto

Ingredients:

- 1 cup Arborio rice

- Four cups of chicken or veggie broth.

- 2 tablespoons olive oil

- 1 onion, finely chopped

- 2 cloves garlic, minced

- 8 ounces of sliced mushrooms (such as cremini or button).

- Add 1/2 cup dry white wine (optional).

- 1/2 cup grated Parmesan cheese

- Salt and pepper to taste

- Fresh parsley for garnish (optional)

Preparation:

1. In a saucepan, heat the chicken or vegetable broth over low heat and keep it warm.

2. In a separate large skillet or saucepan, heat the olive oil over medium heat. Add the chopped onion and garlic, and cook until softened about 3-5 minutes.

3. Cook the sliced mushrooms in the pan until they are soft and browned, approximately 5-7 minutes.

4. Stir in the Arborio rice and cook for 1-2 minutes until the grains are coated with oil and slightly translucent.

5. If using, add the white wine and simmer until absorbed by the rice.

6. Begin adding the warm broth to the rice mixture, one ladleful at a time, stirring frequently. Allow each batch of broth to soak before adding more.

7. Continue adding broth and stirring until the rice is creamy and tender about 20-25 minutes.

8. Stir in the grated Parmesan cheese until melted and creamy.

9. Add salt and pepper to taste.

10. Garnish with fresh parsley if desired and serve hot.

Nutritional Value (per serving):

- Calories: 350

- Total Fat: 10g

- Saturated Fat: 3g

- Cholesterol: 10mg

- Sodium: 800mg

- Total Carbohydrates: 50g

- Dietary Fiber: 3g

- Sugars: 3g

- Protein: 10g

Cooking Time: 35-40 minutes

Number of Servings: 4

6. Sweet and Sour Cabbage

Ingredients:

- One small head of finely sliced green cabbage.

- 1 onion, thinly sliced

- 2 tablespoons vegetable oil

- 1/4 cup apple cider vinegar

- 1/4 cup brown sugar

- 1/4 cup ketchup

- 1 tablespoon soy sauce

- Salt and pepper to taste

Preparation:

1. In a large skillet or wok, heat the vegetable oil over medium heat.

2. Add the sliced onion and cook until softened, about 3-5 minutes.

3. Add the sliced cabbage to the skillet and cook, stirring occasionally, until it begins to wilt, about 5-7 minutes.

4. In a small bowl, whisk together the apple cider vinegar, brown sugar,

ketchup, and soy sauce until well combined.

5. Pour the sauce over the cabbage and onions in the skillet.

6. Reduce the heat to low and simmer, stirring occasionally, until the cabbage is tender and the sauce has thickened, about 15-20 minutes.

7. Add salt and pepper to taste.

8. Serve hot as a side dish.

Nutritional Value (per serving):

- Calories: 120

- Total Fat: 5g

- Sodium: 400mg

- Total Carbohydrates: 18g

- Dietary Fiber: 3g

- Sugars: 13g

- Protein: 2g

Cooking Time: 25-30 minutes

Number of Servings: 4

Ingredients:

- 2 cups cooked rice (ideally a day old).

- 2 tablespoons vegetable oil

- 2 eggs, lightly beaten

- 1 carrot, diced

- 1/2 cup frozen peas, thawed

- 2 green onions, thinly sliced

- 2 tablespoons soy sauce

- 1 tablespoon sesame oil

- Salt and pepper to taste

Preparation:

1. In a large skillet or wok, heat 1 tablespoon vegetable oil over medium heat.

2. Add the beaten eggs to the skillet and scramble until cooked through. Remove from the skillet and put aside.

3. In the same skillet, add the remaining tablespoon of vegetable oil. Add the diced carrot and cook for 2-3 minutes until slightly softened.

4. Add the cooked rice to the skillet, breaking up any clumps, and cook for 3-4 minutes until heated through.

5. Stir in the thawed peas and sliced green onions, and cook for an additional 2-3 minutes.

6. Add the scrambled eggs back to the skillet and drizzle with soy sauce and sesame oil. Stir to combine.

7. Cook for another 1-2 minutes until everything is heated through.

8. Add salt and pepper to taste.

9. Serve hot as a main dish or side.

Nutritional Value (per serving):

- Calories: 280

- Total Fat: 12g

- Saturated Fat: 2g

- Cholesterol: 105mg

- Sodium: 600mg

- Total Carbohydrates: 34g

- Dietary Fiber: 3g

- Sugars: 4g

- Protein: 9g

Cooking Time: 15-20 minutes

Number of Servings: 4

8. Asparagus with Soy and Sesame Mayonnaise

Ingredients:

- 1 pound asparagus, trimmed

- 1/4 cup mayonnaise

- 1 tablespoon soy sauce

- 1 tablespoon sesame oil

- 1 tablespoon sesame seeds, toasted

- Salt and pepper to taste

Preparation:

1. Steam or blanch the asparagus until tender, about 3-5 minutes. Drain and set aside.

2. In a small bowl, whisk together the mayonnaise, soy sauce, and sesame oil until well combined.

3. Arrange the cooked asparagus on a serving platter.

4. Drizzle the soy and sesame mayonnaise mixture over the asparagus.

5. Sprinkle with toasted sesame seeds.

6. Add salt and pepper to taste.

7. Serve immediately.

Nutritional Value (per serving):

- Calories: 150

- Total Fat: 13g

- Saturated Fat: 2g

- Sodium: 400mg

- Total Carbohydrates: 5g

- Dietary Fiber: 2g

- Sugars: 2g

- Protein: 4g

Cooking Time: 10-15 minutes

Number of Servings: 4

CHAPTER 5

1 - Minestrone Soup

Ingredients:

- 2 tablespoons olive oil

- 1 onion, chopped

- 2 cloves garlic, minced

- 2 carrots, diced

- 2 celery stalks, diced

- 1 zucchini, diced

- 1 can (14 oz) diced tomatoes

- 4 cups vegetable broth

- Drain and rinse 1 can (15 oz) of kidney beans.

- One cup of tiny pasta (such as ditalini or macaroni).

- 1 teaspoon dried basil

- 1 teaspoon dried oregano

- Salt and pepper to taste

- Grated Parmesan cheese for serving (optional)

Preparation:

- Sodium: 800mg

1. Heat the olive oil in a big saucepan over medium heat. Sauté the onion and garlic until softened, approximately 5 minutes.

2. Combine the carrots, celery, and zucchini. Cook until the veggies are soft, approximately 7-8 minutes.

3. Stir in diced tomatoes and vegetable broth. Bring to a simmer.

4. Add kidney beans, pasta, basil, and oregano. Simmer for about 10-12 minutes, or until the pasta is done.

5. Add salt and pepper to taste.

6. Serve hot, topped with grated Parmesan cheese if desired.

Nutritional Value:

- Calories: 220

- Total Fat: 5g

- Total Carbohydrates: 35g

- Dietary Fiber: 8g

- Protein: 9g

Cooking Time: Approximately 30 minutes

Servings: 6

2. Cauliflower Soup

Ingredients:

- 1 head cauliflower, chopped into florets
- 2 tablespoons olive oil
- 1 onion, chopped
- 2 cloves garlic, minced
- 4 cups vegetable broth
- 1 cup milk (or non-dairy alternative)
- Salt and pepper to taste
- Fresh parsley for garnish (optional)

Preparation:

1. Preheat oven to 400°F (200°C). Place cauliflower florets on a baking sheet, drizzle with olive oil, and roast for 25-30 minutes, until golden brown.

2. In a big saucepan, heat the olive oil over medium heat. Sauté the onion and garlic until softened, approximately 5 minutes.

3. Combine roasted cauliflower and vegetable broth. Bring to a simmer, and then cook for 15-20 minutes.

4. Use an immersion blender to smooth up the soup. Alternatively, transfer the soup to a blender in stages and process until smooth.

5. Stir in milk and season with salt and pepper to taste.

6. Serve hot, topped with fresh parsley if preferred.

Nutritional Value:

- Calories: 150
- Total Fat: 7g
- Sodium: 700mg
- Total Carbohydrates: 18g
- Dietary Fiber: 5g
- Protein: 6g

Cooking Time: Approximately 1 hour

Servings: 4

3. Lemon Asparagus Soup

Ingredients:

- 1 bunch asparagus, trimmed and chopped

- 2 tablespoons butter

- 1 onion, chopped

- 2 cloves garlic, minced

- 4 cups vegetable broth

- 1 lemon, zest and juice

- 1/2 cup heavy cream (or coconut milk for a dairy-free alternative).

- Salt and pepper to taste

- Fresh chives for garnish (optional)

Preparation:

1. Melt the butter in a large saucepan on medium heat. Sauté the onion and garlic until softened, approximately 5 minutes.

2. Add chopped asparagus and cook for another 5 minutes.

3. Pour in the veggie broth and heat to a boil. Cook the asparagus for 10-12 minutes, or until tender.

4. Use an immersion blender to smooth up the soup. Alternatively, transfer the soup to a blender in stages and process until smooth.

5. Stir in lemon zest, lemon juice, and heavy cream. Season with salt and pepper to taste.

6. Serve hot, topped with fresh chives if preferred.

Nutritional Value:

- Calories: 180

- Total Fat: 14g

- Sodium: 800mg

- Total Carbohydrates: 11g

- Dietary Fiber: 4g

- Protein: 4g

Cooking Time: Approximately 30 minutes

Servings: 4

4. Thai Coconut Soup

Ingredients:

- 1 tablespoon coconut oil
- 1 onion, chopped
- 2 cloves garlic, minced
- 1 red bell pepper, sliced
- 1 tablespoon fresh ginger, grated
- 2 tablespoons Thai red curry paste
- 4 cups vegetable broth
- 1 can (14 oz) coconut milk
- 1 tablespoon soy sauce
- 2 tablespoons lime juice
- 1 tablespoon brown sugar
- Salt to taste
- Fresh cilantro for garnish (optional)

Preparation:

1. In a large saucepan, heat the coconut oil on medium heat. Add onion, garlic, and red bell pepper. Sauté until softened, about 5 minutes.

2. Stir in grated ginger and Thai red curry paste. Cook for another minute.

3. Pour in vegetable broth and coconut milk. Bring to a simmer, then cook for 10 minutes.

4. Add soy sauce, lime juice, and brown sugar. Season with salt to taste.

5. Serve hot, topped with fresh cilantro if preferred.

Nutritional Value:

- Calories: 290
- Total Fat: 24g
- Sodium: 900mg
- Total Carbohydrates: 15g
- Dietary Fiber: 2g
- Protein: 4g

Cooking Time: Approximately 30 minutes

Servings: 4

Ingredients:

- Cut one pound of white fish fillets (such as cod or haddock) into pieces.

- 2 tablespoons butter

- 1 onion, chopped

- 2 cloves garlic, minced

- 2 potatoes, peeled and diced

- 4 cups fish or vegetable broth

- 1 cup milk

- 1/4 cup all-purpose flour

- Zest and juice of 1 lemon

- 2 tablespoons fresh dill, chopped

- Salt and pepper to taste

Preparation:

1. In a big saucepan, melt the butter on medium heat. Sauté the onion and garlic for 5 minutes, or until they are softened.

2. Add diced potatoes and cook for another 5 minutes.

3. Sprinkle flour over the veggies and toss to mix.

4. Gradually pour in fish or vegetable broth, stirring constantly to avoid lumps.

5. Add fish chunks to the pot and bring to a simmer. Cook until fish is cooked through and potatoes are tender about 10-12 minutes.

6. In a small bowl, whisk together milk and lemon zest. Pour into the saucepan and mix thoroughly.

7. Add lemon juice and fresh dill. Season with salt and pepper to taste.

8. Serve hot.

Nutritional Value:

- Calories: 300

- Total Fat: 9g

- Sodium: 700mg

- Total Carbohydrates: 32g

- Dietary Fiber: 3g

- Protein: 24g

Cooking Time: Approximately 30 minutes

Servings: 4

6. Mexican Tortilla Soup

Ingredients:

- 1 tablespoon olive oil

- 1 onion, chopped

- 2 cloves garlic, minced

- 1 red bell pepper, chopped

- 1 jalapeño pepper, seeded and diced

- 1 can (14 oz) diced tomatoes

- 4 cups chicken or vegetable broth

- 1 teaspoon ground cumin

- 1 teaspoon chili powder

- Salt and pepper to taste

- Tortilla strips, avocado slices, shredded cheese, and chopped cilantro for garnish

Preparation:

1. Warm the olive oil in a big saucepan over medium heat. Combine onions, garlic, red bell pepper, and jalapeño pepper. Sauté for about 5 minutes, or until softened. Sauté until softened, about 5 minutes.

2. Stir in diced tomatoes, chicken or vegetable broth, ground cumin, and chili powder. Simmer for 15-20 minutes.

3. Sprinkle with salt and pepper as desired.

4. Serve hot, garnished with tortilla strips, avocado slices, shredded cheese, and chopped cilantro.

Nutritional Value:

- Calories: 180

- Total Fat: 8g

- Sodium: 800mg

- Total Carbohydrates: 24g

- Dietary Fiber: 5g

- Protein: 6g

Cooking Time: Approximately 30 minutes

Servings: 4

7. Tomato Basil Soup

Ingredients:

- 2 tablespoons olive oil

- 1 onion, chopped

- 2 cloves garlic, minced

- 2 cans (14 oz each) diced tomatoes

- 4 cups vegetable broth

- 1/2 cup fresh basil leaves, chopped

- 1/2 cup heavy cream (optional)

- Salt and pepper to taste

- Grated Parmesan cheese for garnish (optional)

Preparation:

1. Warm the olive oil in a big saucepan over medium heat. Sauté the onion and garlic for 5 minutes, or until they are softened.

2. Add diced tomatoes and vegetable broth. Simmer for 15-20 minutes.

3. Add in the chopped basil leaves. To make the soup smooth, use an immersion blender. Alternatively, put the soup in a blender and process it in batches until smooth.

4. Stir in heavy cream (if using) and season with salt and pepper to taste.

5. Serve hot, with optional grated Parmesan cheese.

Nutritional Value:

- Calories: 180

- Total Fat: 10g

- Sodium: 800mg

- Total Carbohydrates: 16g

- Dietary Fiber: 4g

- Protein: 3g

Cooking Time: Approximately 30 minutes

Servings: 4

8. Spinach Lentil Soup

Ingredients:

- 1 tablespoon olive oil

- 1 onion, chopped

- 2 cloves garlic, minced

- 1 carrot, diced

- 1 celery stalk, diced

- Rinsed and drained 1 cup dry lentils.

- 4 cups vegetable broth

- 2 cups fresh spinach leaves

- 1 teaspoon ground cumin

- Salt and pepper to taste

- Lemon wedges for serving (optional)

Preparation:

1. Warm the olive oil in a big saucepan over medium heat. Sauté the onion and garlic for 5 minutes, or until they are softened.

2. Add diced carrots and celery. Cook for another 5 minutes.

3. Stir in dried lentils and vegetable broth. Bring to a simmer and cook for 20-25 minutes, or until lentils are tender.

4. Add fresh spinach leaves and ground cumin. Cook for about 2-3 minutes, or until the spinach has wilted.

5. Season with salt and pepper as desired.

6. Serve hot, with lemon wedges for squeezing over the soup if desired.

Nutritional Value:

-   Calories: 220

-   Total Fat: 4g

-   Sodium: 800mg

-   Total Carbohydrates: 32g

-   Dietary Fiber: 16g

-   Protein: 12g

Cooking Time: Approximately 45 minutes

Servings: 4

CHAPTER 6

1. Lemon Sorbet

Ingredients:

- 1 cup freshly squeezed lemon juice

- 1 cup water

- 1 cup granulated sugar

Preparation:

1. In a saucepan, combine water and sugar over medium heat. Stir until the sugar dissolves completely to make a simple syrup.

2. Turn off the heat and let it cool to a comfortable level.

3. Stir in freshly squeezed lemon juice into the simple syrup.

4. Transfer the mixture to an ice cream machine and churn according to the manufacturer's directions until it reaches sorbet consistency.

5. Transfer the sorbet to a freezer-safe container and freeze for at least 4 hours before serving.

Nutritional Value: Each serving (1/2 cup) contains approximately 110 calories, 0g fat, 28g carbohydrates, and 0g protein.

Cooking Time: Approximately 10 minutes (excluding freezing time).

Servings: 6 servings.

2. Chia Seed Pudding

Ingredients:

- 1/4 cup chia seeds

- 1 cup almond milk (or other milk of your preference).

- One spoonful of honey or maple syrup (optional).

- Fresh fruits or nuts for topping (optional)

Preparation:

1. In a bowl, mix chia seeds, almond milk, and honey or maple syrup (if using). Stir well.

2. Cover the dish and chill for at least 2 hours, preferably overnight, to enable the chia seeds to absorb the liquid and thicken.

3. Stir the pudding mixture before serving and add desired toppings like fresh fruits or nuts.

Nutritional Value: Each serving contains approximately 150 calories, 8g fat, 15g carbohydrates, 5g protein.

Cooking Time: 5 minutes preparation + chilling time.

Servings: 2 servings.

3. Almond Flour Cookies

Ingredients:

- 2 cups almond flour

- Use 1/4 cup melted coconut oil or butter.

- 1/4 cup honey or maple syrup.

- 1 teaspoon vanilla extract

- 1/4 teaspoon baking soda

- Pinch of salt

Preparation:

1. Heat the oven to 350°F (175°C) and prepare a baking sheet with parchment paper.

2. In a bowl, mix almond flour, melted coconut oil or butter, honey or maple syrup, vanilla extract, baking soda, and salt until well combined.

3. Scoop tablespoon-sized portions of dough and roll into balls. Place them on the prepared baking sheet and gently flatten with your hand.

4. Bake for 10-12 minutes or until the edges are golden brown.

5. Allow the cookies to cool on the baking sheet for 5 minutes before transferring to a wire rack to cool completely.

Nutritional Value: Each cookie contains approximately 120 calories, 10g fat, 6g carbohydrates, and 3g protein.

Cooking Time: Approximately 12 minutes.

Servings: 12 cookies.

4. Baked Apple Slices

Ingredients:

- Two big apples, cored and thinly sliced

- 1 tablespoon lemon juice

- 1 teaspoon ground cinnamon

- One spoonful of maple syrup or honey (optional).

Preparation:

1. Heat the oven to 350°F (175°C) and prepare a baking sheet with parchment paper.

2. In a large bowl, toss the apple slices with lemon juice, ground cinnamon, and honey or maple syrup (if using) until evenly coated.

3. Arrange the apple slices in a single layer on the prepared baking sheet.

4. Bake for 20-25 minutes or until the apples are tender and slightly caramelized.

5. Serve warm as is or with a dollop of yogurt or a sprinkle of granola, if desired.

Nutritional Value: Each serving contains approximately 60 calories, 0g fat, 16g carbohydrates, and 0g protein.

Cooking Time: Approximately 25 minutes.

Servings: 4 servings.

5. Vanilla Almond Bites

Ingredients:

- 1 cup almond flour

- Two spoonful of maple syrup or honey.

- 1 teaspoon vanilla extract

- Pinch of salt

- Optional toppings include melted chocolate, chopped nuts, and shredded coconut.

Preparation:

1. In a mixing bowl, combine almond flour, honey or maple syrup, vanilla extract, and a pinch of salt. Mix until a dough forms.

2. Roll the dough into small bite-sized balls and place them on a plate or baking sheet lined with parchment paper.

3. If desired, roll the bites in optional toppings like melted chocolate, chopped nuts, or shredded coconut.

4. Refrigerate the bites for at least 30 minutes to firm up before serving.

Nutritional Value: Each bite contains approximately 50 calories, 3g fat, 5g carbohydrates, and 1g protein.

Cooking Time: 10 minutes preparation + chilling time.

Servings: 12 bites.

6. Raspberry Frozen Yogurt

Ingredients:

- 2 cups frozen raspberries

- 2 cups plain Greek yogurt

- 1/4 cup honey or maple syrup (optional, adjust to taste)

Preparation:

1. In a blender or food processor, combine frozen raspberries, Greek yogurt, and honey or maple syrup (if using).

2. Blend until smooth and creamy.

3. Taste and adjust the sweetness as needed by adding additional honey or maple syrup.

4. Place the mixture in a freezer-safe container and freeze for at least 4 hours, or until hard.

5. Allow the frozen yogurt to soften slightly at room temperature for a few minutes before serving.

Nutritional Value: Each serving contains approximately 120 calories, 0g fat, 20g carbohydrates, 10g protein.

Cooking Time: 5 minutes preparation + freezing time.

Servings: 4 servings.

7. Blueberry Protein Bites

Ingredients:

- 1 cup rolled oats

- Half a cup of almond or peanut butter.

- 1/4 cup of maple syrup or honey.

- 1/4 cup unflavored or vanilla protein powder.

- 1/2 cup dried blueberries

- 1/4 cup unsweetened shredded coconut

Preparation:

1. In a food processor, blend rolled oats until finely ground.

2. Add almond butter or peanut butter, honey or maple syrup, protein powder, dried blueberries, and shredded coconut to the food processor. Blend until the mixture comes together and forms dough.

3. If the mixture is too dry, add a tablespoon of water at a time until it reaches a dough-like consistency.

4. Scoop tablespoon-sized portions of the dough and roll into balls.

5. Place the balls on a plate or baking sheet lined with parchment paper and refrigerate for at least 30 minutes to firm up.

Nutritional Value: *Each bite contains approximately 90 calories, 4g fat, 11g carbohydrates, and 4g protein.*

Cooking Time: *10 minutes preparation + chilling time.*

Servings: *12 bites.*

8. Baked Apple Slices (variation)

Ingredients:

- Two big apples, cored and finely sliced.

- 1 tablespoon lemon juice

- 1 teaspoon ground cinnamon

- 1 tablespoon honey or maple syrup

- 1/4 cup almond slices or chopped walnuts (optional)

Preparation:

1. Preheat the oven to 375°F (190°C) and grease a baking dish with cooking spray or butter.

2. In a bowl, toss the apple slices with lemon juice, ground cinnamon, and honey or maple syrup until evenly coated.

3. Arrange the apple slices in the greased baking dish. Sprinkle almond slices or chopped walnuts on top, if using.

4. Bake for 25-30 minutes or until the apples are tender and the topping is golden brown.

5. Serve warm as is or with a scoop of vanilla ice cream for a decadent treat.

Nutritional Value: Each serving contains approximately 80 calories, 2g fat, 18g carbohydrates, 1g protein.

Cooking Time: Approximately 30 minutes.

Servings: 4 servings.

CONCLUSION

In conclusion, this Type 2 Diabetes Cookbook for Beginners 2024 serves as an invaluable resource for individuals navigating the challenges of managing diabetes through dietary interventions. Throughout this cookbook, we've explored a plethora of delicious and nutritious recipes tailored specifically to support stable blood sugar levels and overall well-being. From breakfast to dinner, snacks to desserts, each recipe has been meticulously crafted to strike the perfect balance between flavor and health.

Moreover, beyond just providing recipes, this cookbook has sought to empower readers with knowledge about the role of nutrition in managing type 2 diabetes. By understanding the impact of different foods on blood sugar levels and incorporating mindful eating habits, readers are equipped with the tools to make informed dietary choices that can positively influence their health outcomes.

As we conclude this journey through the pages of this cookbook, it's important to recognize that adopting a healthy diet for managing type 2 diabetes is not merely about restriction, but about abundance. Embracing a diverse array of nutrient-rich foods not only supports optimal blood sugar control but also fosters a sense of culinary exploration and enjoyment.

To the reader, I offer a special motivation: Embrace this cookbook not as a rigid set of rules, but as a blueprint for crafting a lifestyle that honors your health and vitality. See each recipe as an opportunity to nourish your body with wholesome ingredients that fuel your well-being. Approach every meal with curiosity and creativity, knowing that you have the power to transform your health through the simple act of cooking.

As you embark on this culinary journey, remember that small changes can yield significant results. Celebrate your successes, learn from setbacks, and above all, be kind to yourself along the way. With dedication, patience, and a dash of culinary flair, you can thrive on this journey toward better health and well-being. Cheers to delicious meals, vibrant health, and a brighter future ahead!

BONUS

Day 1:

- Breakfast: cottage cheese, sliced peaches, and cinnamon.

- Lunch: Grilled chicken salad with mixed greens, tomatoes, cucumbers, and vinaigrette dressing

- Dinner: Baked salmon with roasted vegetables (broccoli, cauliflower, and carrots) and quinoa

Day 2:

- Breakfast: A veggie omelet with spinach, bell peppers, and onions.

- Lunch: Wrap with turkey and avocado on whole wheat tortillas.

- Dinner: Stir-fried tofu with bell peppers, snap peas, and brown rice

Day 3:

- Breakfast: Overnight oats made with rolled oats, almond milk, chia seeds, and sliced banana

- Lunch: Lentil soup with whole grain bread.

- Dinner: Grilled shrimp skewers with grilled zucchini and couscous.

Day 4:

- Breakfast: Whole grain toast with avocado spread and sliced tomatoes

- Lunch: Quinoa salad with chickpeas, cherry tomatoes, cucumbers, and feta cheese.

- Dinner: Baked chicken breast with steamed broccoli and sweet potato

Day 5:

- Breakfast: Smoothie prepared with spinach, banana, almond milk, and protein powder.

- Lunch: Black bean and vegetable burrito bowl with salsa and guacamole.

- Dinner: Beef stir fry with bell peppers, onions, and brown rice.

Day 6:

- Breakfast: Cottage cheese topped with sliced peaches and honey.

- Lunch: Grilled veggie and hummus wrap with whole wheat tortillas.

- Dinner: Baked cod with asparagus and quinoa pilaf

Day 7:

- Breakfast: scrambled eggs, sautéed mushrooms, and whole grain bread.

- Lunch: Spinach salad with grilled chicken, strawberries, almonds, and balsamic vinaigrette

- Dinner: Turkey meatballs with marinara sauce over whole wheat spaghetti.

Day 8:

- Breakfast: Plain Greek yogurt topped with sliced apple and a sprinkle of cinnamon

- Lunch: Tuna salad made with canned tuna, mixed greens, cherry tomatoes, and lemon vinaigrette

- Dinner: Baked tofu with roasted Brussels sprouts and quinoa

Day 9:

- Breakfast: Whole grain English muffin with scrambled eggs and avocado slices

- Lunch: Chickpeas and vegetable curry with brown rice.

- Dinner: Grilled steak with steamed green beans and a baked sweet potato

Day 10:

- Breakfast: Protein smoothie made with spinach, mixed berries, almond milk, and protein powder

- Lunch: Stir-fried turkey and vegetables with quinoa.

- Dinner: Baked salmon with roasted asparagus and wild rice

Day 11:

- Breakfast: Oatmeal topped with sliced banana, chopped walnuts, and a drizzle of honey.

- Lunch: A Caesar salad with romaine lettuce, grilled chicken breast, Parmesan cheese, and Caesar dressing.

- Dinner: Lentil and vegetable stew with wholesome bread.

Day 12:

- Breakfast: Whole-grain bread with almond butter and cut strawberries.

- Lunch: Veggie and hummus wrap with whole wheat tortilla

- Dinner: Grilled shrimp with mixed greens salad and a side of quinoa

Day 13:

- Breakfast: egg scramble with sautéed spinach and tomatoes.

- Lunch: Quinoa salad tossed with black beans, corn, sliced bell peppers, and lime vinaigrette.

- Dinner: Baked chicken thighs with roasted cauliflower and brown rice

Day 14:

- Breakfast: Cottage cheese with pineapple chunks and a sprinkle of shredded coconut

- Lunch: turkey and avocado sandwich on whole grain toast with a side salad.

- Dinner: Tofu stir-fried with broccoli, bell peppers, and brown rice.

Day 15:

- Breakfast: Smoothie bowl topped with sliced banana, granola, and a drizzle of honey

- Lunch: Spinach and feta stuffed chicken breast with roasted vegetables

- Dinner: Lentil and vegetable stir-fry with brown rice

Day 16:

- Breakfast: Whole grain English muffin with scrambled eggs and smoked salmon

- Lunch: Quinoa and black bean salad with diced tomatoes, avocado, and cilantro-lime dressing

- Dinner: Grilled pork chops with steamed broccoli and quinoa pilaf

Day 17:

- Breakfast: Greek yogurt parfait with layers of granola and mixed berries

- Lunch: Turkey and vegetable stir-fry with tofu noodles

- Dinner: Baked fish with roasted Brussels sprouts and sweet potato mash.

Day 18:

- Breakfast: Whole grain toast with almond butter and sliced pear

- Lunch: Chicken and vegetable soup with a side of whole grain bread

- Dinner: Beef and broccoli stir-fry with brown rice

Day 19:

- Breakfast: Overnight oats made with rolled oats, almond milk, chia seeds, and diced mango

- Lunch: Spinach salad with grilled chicken, strawberries, almonds, and balsamic vinaigrette

- Dinner: Turkey meatballs in marinara sauce served over spaghetti squash.

Day 20:

- Breakfast: Veggie omelet with mushrooms, bell peppers, onions, and feta cheese

- Lunch: Lentil and vegetable wrap with whole wheat tortilla

- Dinner: Grilled shrimp skewers with mixed greens salad and quinoa

Day 21:

- Breakfast: cottage cheese topped with sliced peaches and cinnamon.

- Lunch: Tuna salad lettuce wraps stuffed with avocado and cherry tomatoes.

- Dinner: Baked tofu with roasted cauliflower and wild rice.

Day 22:

- Breakfast: A protein smoothie with spinach, banana, almond milk, and protein powder.

- Lunch: Turkey and avocado salad with mixed greens, cucumber, and a light vinaigrette dressing

- Dinner: Salmon grilled with asparagus and quinoa.

Day 23:

- Breakfast: Whole grain bread with mashed avocado and sliced tomatoes.

- Lunch: Quinoa and black bean burrito bowl with salsa, guacamole, and Greek yogurt.

- Dinner: Baked chicken breast, steaming green beans, brown rice.

Day 24:

- Breakfast: Oatmeal topped with sliced banana, chopped nuts, and a drizzle of maple syrup

- Lunch: Chickpea and vegetable stir-fry with tofu and brown rice

- Dinner: Beef and veggie kebabs served with couscous.

Day 25:

- Breakfast: Greek yogurt with mixed berries and a sprinkle of granola

- Lunch: Turkey and vegetable wrap with hummus and whole wheat tortilla

- Dinner: baked fish with roasted Brussels sprouts and quinoa pilaf.

Day 26:

- Breakfast: Smoothie made with spinach, pineapple, Greek yogurt, and almond milk

- Lunch: Lentil soup and whole grain toast.

- Dinner: Grilled shrimp with mixed greens salad and a side of sweet potato

Day 27:

- Breakfast: Whole grain English muffin with scrambled eggs and spinach

- Lunch: turkey and avocado sandwich on whole grain bread, along with carrot sticks.

- Dinner: Tofu stir-fried with broccoli, bell peppers, and brown rice.

Day 28:

- Breakfast: Cottage cheese with sliced mango and a sprinkle of coconut flakes.

- Lunch: Spinach and feta-filled chicken breast served with roasted veggies.

- Dinner: Lentil and vegetable curry with quinoa